Table of Contents

Chapter 1: Understanding Repurposed Drugs for Cancer

Chapter 2: Metformin – A Metabolic Disruptor in Cancer Therapy

Chapter 3: Types of Cancer Metformin May Help Prevent and Treat

Chapter 4: Low-Dose Naltrexone (LDN) and Immunomodulation

Chapter 5: Statins, Antibiotics, and Blood Thinners – Surprising Anti-Cancer Agents

Chapter 6: Practical Protocols and Future Directions

Chapter 1: Understanding Repurposed Drugs in Cancer Therapy

A New Approach to Cancer Treatment

For decades, cancer treatment has centered around three main approaches—surgery, chemotherapy, and radiation. While these methods have saved lives, they often come with limitations, including harsh side effects, tumor resistance, and recurrence. As researchers continue to search for better solutions, an unexpected avenue has gained attention: the use of **existing, FDA-approved drugs** for treating cancer.

Repurposed drugs—medications originally designed for other conditions but now showing promise in cancer treatment—offer a **new way to target cancer metabolism, inflammation, and immune response**. These drugs are already widely available, have known safety profiles, and, in many cases, cost a fraction of new cancer drugs. Scientists have begun to recognize that certain medications, from diabetes drugs to anti-parasitics, may hold the **key to slowing**

tumor growth, enhancing treatment response, and even preventing cancer in high-risk individuals.

Why Repurposing Drugs Matters

The development of new cancer treatments is slow and expensive. Traditional drug discovery can take over a decade, with only a small percentage of new drugs ever making it to market. In contrast, repurposed drugs have already been tested for safety in humans, making them a faster and more cost-effective option.

Beyond the practicality of using existing medications, these drugs offer something even more valuable—a way to **disrupt the metabolic and immune pathways that cancer depends on**. Instead of attacking tumors directly, some of these drugs weaken cancer's support system, cutting off its fuel supply, interfering with growth signals, and making it more vulnerable to standard treatments. Others work by reducing inflammation, enhancing the immune system, or stopping the formation of new blood vessels that feed tumors.

This shift in thinking is leading to new possibilities. Research has revealed that certain widely used drugs—including metformin, ivermectin, low-dose naltrexone, and statins—may be able to **alter the internal environment of the body in ways that make it harder for cancer to thrive**. Scientists and clinicians are now studying these medications in clinical trials, hoping to refine protocols and determine the best ways to integrate them into cancer care.

Repurposed drugs are not meant to replace conventional cancer treatments, but they may complement them in ways that improve survival rates and quality of life. They offer a practical, accessible option that gives patients and doctors more tools in the fight against cancer. With an increasing body of research supporting their use, it is becoming clear that **drug repurposing is not just a possibility— it is an emerging frontier in cancer therapy**.

Why Existing Drugs Are Being Explored for Cancer

The idea of repurposing medications for cancer treatment isn't just about convenience—it's about necessity. Despite billions of dollars spent on new drug development, cancer remains one of the most complex and challenging diseases to treat. Traditional therapies often struggle with two major problems: resistance and recurrence. Even when a treatment appears successful, cancer can adapt, finding new pathways to grow and spread. This has led researchers to explore existing drugs that might **disrupt cancer's survival mechanisms in unexpected ways**.

One of the biggest advantages of repurposed drugs is their **established safety profile**. Unlike new drugs that require years of testing, these medications have already been used for other conditions, meaning doctors understand their risks, side effects, and interactions. This allows researchers to move directly into clinical trials that assess their effectiveness against cancer, rather than spending years determining whether they are safe for human use.

Another factor driving interest in repurposed drugs is **cost**. The development of new cancer medications is incredibly expensive, often exceeding a billion dollars per drug. These costs are passed down to patients, making cutting-edge treatments financially out of reach for many. Repurposed drugs, on the other hand, are often **off-patent and inexpensive**, meaning they could provide **affordable cancer-fighting options** for a larger population.

How Cancer Metabolism Can Be Targeted with Repurposed Drugs

Cancer is more than just uncontrolled cell division. It is a **metabolic disease**, meaning tumors rely on specific energy sources and biochemical pathways to grow. Unlike healthy cells, which can efficiently switch between using carbohydrates, fats, and proteins for energy, cancer cells are **highly**

dependent on glucose and insulin signaling to fuel their rapid expansion. This is one of the reasons why people with insulin resistance or diabetes often have a higher risk of developing certain cancers.

Many repurposed drugs work by **interfering with these metabolic pathways**, depriving cancer of its preferred fuel. Metformin, for example, lowers insulin and blood sugar levels, reducing the availability of energy for tumor cells. Statins, originally designed to lower cholesterol, also disrupt cancer metabolism by interfering with the production of compounds that cancer cells need to build new membranes.

Beyond metabolism, some repurposed drugs **target inflammation and immune function**, two factors that play a major role in cancer progression. Chronic inflammation creates an environment where cancer thrives, while a weakened immune system allows tumors to evade detection. Drugs like low-dose naltrexone help regulate immune responses, potentially making it easier for the body to recognize and eliminate cancerous cells.

As researchers continue to test repurposed drugs, a clearer picture is emerging—one where **targeting cancer's weaknesses through metabolic and immune disruption may be just as important as directly attacking tumors with chemotherapy or radiation**.

How Cancer Metabolism and Growth Pathways Can Be Disrupted

Cancer is often thought of as a genetic disease—something that happens when mutations occur in cells, causing them to grow uncontrollably. While genetic changes do play a role, many researchers now recognize that cancer is also deeply **linked to metabolism**. Unlike normal cells, which follow strict rules for energy use and division, cancer cells **rewire their metabolism** to sustain continuous growth. This shift in energy use is known as the **Warburg effect**, a process where cancer cells prefer fermenting glucose for energy, even when oxygen is available.

This metabolic reliance on glucose means that cancer cells are highly **sensitive to changes in insulin levels, nutrient availability, and cellular energy balance**. Many repurposed drugs work by interfering with these pathways, depriving tumors of the resources they need to grow. Metformin, for example, lowers blood sugar and activates **AMPK**, an energy-sensing enzyme that forces cells into a more energy-efficient state. Since cancer thrives on high energy availability, activating AMPK can make it harder for tumors to expand.

Growth Pathways That Repurposed Drugs Can Target

Beyond metabolism, cancer cells use several key growth pathways to multiply and spread. Two of the most well-studied pathways in cancer research are **mTOR (mechanistic target of rapamycin) and IGF-1 (insulin-like growth factor-1)**. These pathways act as **growth signals**, telling cells when to divide and when to build new proteins. In normal cells, these signals are carefully regulated, but in cancer cells, they are often overactive.

Certain repurposed drugs are known to **suppress these pathways**, slowing down tumor progression. Statins, for instance, interfere with cholesterol synthesis, but they also inhibit important signaling molecules involved in cancer growth. Metformin reduces IGF-1 levels, making it harder for tumors to receive the **constant stimulation they need to keep dividing**.

Other repurposed drugs, such as ivermectin, work by **disrupting cellular communication** in tumors. Some cancers rely on the **WNT pathway**, a network of signals that help cells grow, migrate, and resist treatment. Ivermectin has been shown to block this pathway in some cancers, making it a potential tool for weakening tumors that are resistant to chemotherapy.

These findings suggest that rather than treating cancer as a purely genetic disease, an effective approach may be to **disrupt the**

metabolic and biochemical conditions that allow it to thrive. By cutting off its fuel supply, blocking its growth signals, and making it more vulnerable to the immune system, repurposed drugs may offer a powerful **multi-pronged attack against cancer**.

Historical Examples of Repurposed Drugs Becoming Mainstream Cancer Treatments

The idea of using existing drugs for new medical purposes isn't new. Many of today's most well-known cancer treatments **started as medications for entirely different conditions** before scientists discovered their unexpected anti-cancer effects. These historical examples prove that drug repurposing is not just theoretical—it is a strategy that has already saved lives.

One of the best-known cases is **thalidomide**, a drug that was initially prescribed in the 1950s as a treatment for morning sickness. While it was later banned due to birth defects, researchers discovered that it had powerful effects on **blood vessel formation and the immune system**. Today, thalidomide and its derivatives are **key treatments for multiple myeloma**, a type of blood cancer, because they help suppress tumor blood supply and boost immune response.

Another example is **aspirin**, a simple pain reliever that has been used for over a century. Researchers later discovered that aspirin can **reduce inflammation and inhibit the COX-2 enzyme**, which plays a role in tumor growth. Long-term studies have shown that people who take low-dose aspirin regularly have **a lower risk of developing colorectal cancer**, leading to its inclusion in some cancer prevention protocols.

Statins, originally designed to **lower cholesterol**, were never intended to treat cancer, yet their ability to **block cellular growth pathways and reduce inflammation** has made them an area of active research in oncology. Some studies suggest that statins may **slow tumor progression and enhance**

the effectiveness of chemotherapy, especially in breast and prostate cancers.

The Shift in Thinking About Cancer Treatments

These discoveries have forced scientists to **rethink how cancer is treated**. Instead of focusing only on developing new, highly targeted drugs, there is now increasing interest in finding **existing, affordable medications** that may already hold the answers. Many of these drugs are off-patent, making them inexpensive compared to new cancer drugs that cost **hundreds of thousands of dollars per year**.

More importantly, repurposed drugs offer a **different approach** to cancer treatment. Instead of directly attacking cancer cells—an approach that often leads to resistance—they **alter the body's internal environment** to make it harder for cancer to grow in the first place. This includes:

- **Lowering insulin and glucose levels**, reducing cancer's access to fuel.

- **Suppressing inflammation**, which creates a pro-cancer environment.
- **Modulating the immune system**, making it easier for the body to fight tumors naturally.

This shift in thinking is driving a **new wave of clinical research**, where scientists are systematically testing common drugs to see which ones have unexpected cancer-fighting properties. With each new discovery, it becomes clearer that the next breakthrough in cancer treatment may not come from a new laboratory invention, but from **a drug that has been sitting on pharmacy shelves for years**.

The First Links Between Metformin and Cancer Prevention

One of the earliest repurposed drugs to gain serious attention for its potential anti-cancer effects was **metformin**, a medication long used to manage type 2 diabetes. While metformin's ability to lower blood sugar and improve insulin sensitivity has been well understood for decades, its potential role in

reducing cancer risk was discovered almost by accident.

Doctors began noticing an unusual pattern—diabetic patients taking metformin seemed to develop cancer at **lower rates** compared to those on other diabetes medications. This was first observed in **large-scale population studies**, where researchers found that diabetics on metformin had a significantly **lower incidence of several cancers**, including breast, colorectal, and pancreatic cancer. The protective effect was strong enough to spark deeper investigation into what was happening at a cellular level.

Why Scientists Took Notice

What made these findings so compelling was that the reduced cancer risk **wasn't just a result of better blood sugar control**. Many diabetes drugs lower glucose, but only metformin showed a consistent **cancer-protective effect**. This suggested that metformin was doing something beyond simply improving metabolism—it was directly influencing the biological pathways that cancer relies on.

Further research uncovered several mechanisms that could explain metformin's impact on cancer:

- **Lowering insulin and IGF-1 levels** – Cancer cells thrive in environments with **high insulin and growth factor activity**. By reducing these signals, metformin makes it harder for tumors to receive the stimulation they need to grow.
- **Activating AMPK (AMP-activated protein kinase)** – AMPK acts as a **cellular energy sensor**, signaling cells to conserve energy. Since cancer cells require high energy levels to divide rapidly, metformin's activation of AMPK forces them into an **energy-restricted state**, making it harder for them to grow.
- **Suppressing the mTOR pathway** – The mTOR pathway is a master regulator of cell growth and proliferation. Many

aggressive cancers have **overactive mTOR signaling**, but metformin has been shown to inhibit this pathway, slowing tumor progression.

These discoveries positioned metformin as one of the **first major examples** of a widely used drug that **was never designed to fight cancer but seemed to do so anyway**. As scientists continued to test metformin in animal studies and clinical trials, more evidence emerged that it could **not only reduce cancer risk but also improve outcomes for patients already undergoing treatment**.

Metformin's story is just one example of how **repurposed drugs are challenging the way we think about cancer therapy**. The realization that an inexpensive diabetes medication could have such profound effects on cancer biology **opened the door for further research** into other existing drugs—some of which may be just as promising.

Chapter 2: The Science Behind Metformin and Cancer

How Cancer Cells Thrive – A Look at Their Metabolic Needs

Cancer is often thought of as a disease of uncontrolled cell division, but at its core, it is also a **metabolic disorder**. Unlike healthy cells, which efficiently use oxygen to produce energy through the mitochondria, many cancer cells rely on an alternative process called **aerobic glycolysis**, also known as the **Warburg effect**.

This means that, even when oxygen is available, cancer cells prefer to **ferment glucose for energy**, a process that is far less efficient but allows for **rapid growth and survival under stress**. This shift in metabolism is not just a side effect of cancer—it is a key driver of its progression. Tumors manipulate their environment to ensure a constant supply of **glucose, insulin, and growth factors**, which fuels their ability to expand, invade, and resist treatment.

The Role of Insulin and IGF-1 in Cancer Growth

One of the most significant findings in cancer research is that **high insulin levels and insulin-like growth factor-1 (IGF-1) accelerate tumor progression**. These hormones act as powerful growth signals, instructing cells to take in nutrients and divide. In individuals with **insulin resistance, metabolic syndrome, or diabetes**, insulin and IGF-1 levels are often elevated, creating a **pro-cancer environment** where tumors receive **an excess of fuel and growth stimulation**.

Certain cancers, including **breast, prostate, colorectal, and pancreatic cancer**, are particularly responsive to insulin and IGF-1. Their cells **overexpress insulin receptors**, making them even more sensitive to growth signals. This is why people with **poor metabolic health** tend to have a **higher risk of developing aggressive cancers**.

By lowering **insulin and IGF-1 levels**, it becomes possible to **starve cancer of the**

metabolic support it relies on. This is where **metformin enters the picture**—it reduces blood sugar, improves insulin sensitivity, and helps bring these growth signals back to normal levels.

Research has shown that metformin **not only reduces the likelihood of developing cancer in high-risk individuals but may also slow the progression of existing tumors**. This has led to increasing interest in using metformin as a **preventative measure** for those with metabolic disorders and as a **supportive therapy for patients already battling cancer**.

By shifting cancer cells into an energy-restricted state and cutting off their preferred fuel supply, metformin **weakens their ability to multiply**, setting the stage for further research into how it can be combined with other treatments to improve outcomes.

How Metformin Disrupts Cancer Growth

Metformin's ability to influence cancer isn't a coincidence—it directly targets the metabolic and growth pathways that tumors rely on to survive. Unlike traditional chemotherapy, which aims to kill cancer cells outright, metformin works by **changing the conditions that allow cancer to thrive**, making it harder for tumors to grow and spread.

One of metformin's most significant effects is its role in **reducing glucose and insulin levels**. Cancer cells are highly dependent on **a constant supply of sugar and growth signals** to sustain their rapid division. By improving insulin sensitivity and lowering circulating insulin, metformin helps cut off one of the tumor's primary fuel sources. This is particularly important for cancers that **overexpress insulin receptors**, such as those found in the **breast, prostate, pancreas, and colon**.

Beyond insulin regulation, metformin also exerts its **anti-cancer effects through AMPK activation**. AMPK (AMP-activated protein kinase) is an energy-sensing enzyme that acts as a **metabolic master switch**.

When AMPK is activated, cells shift into an **energy-conserving state**, slowing growth and reducing unnecessary energy consumption. Cancer cells, which require **high metabolic activity to sustain uncontrolled division**, struggle under these conditions.

AMPK and the Cellular Energy Crisis in Tumors

The activation of AMPK forces cells to **prioritize survival over growth**, which is the opposite of what cancer needs. When AMPK is switched on, it:

- **Lowers glucose uptake**, depriving cancer cells of their preferred fuel.
- **Reduces fat and protein synthesis**, limiting the raw materials needed for tumor expansion.
- **Inhibits cell proliferation**, slowing down the rapid division that defines cancer.

This energy crisis creates a **hostile environment for tumor cells**, making them weaker and more vulnerable to stress. Research suggests that metformin-induced

AMPK activation may even help enhance the effects of **chemotherapy and radiation**, making them more effective at destroying cancer cells.

The connection between metformin and cancer metabolism has led to **clinical trials testing metformin in combination with standard treatments**, particularly in cancers that are linked to **insulin resistance and metabolic dysfunction**. These findings are pushing scientists to rethink the role of **metabolic interventions in cancer therapy**, recognizing that the body's internal environment plays a much larger role in cancer progression than previously thought.

Metformin and Apoptosis – Triggering Cancer Cell Death

One of the key challenges in treating cancer is that tumor cells **evade the normal mechanisms of programmed cell death**, a process known as **apoptosis**. In healthy cells, apoptosis acts as a built-in safeguard, ensuring that damaged or unneeded cells self-destruct before they can cause harm. Cancer, however, overrides this system, allowing malignant cells to continue dividing unchecked.

Metformin has been shown to **restore apoptotic signaling**, making it harder for cancer cells to resist destruction. This effect is particularly important for tumors that have become resistant to **chemotherapy and radiation**, as these treatments often rely on triggering apoptosis to shrink tumors.

Research suggests that metformin induces apoptosis in several ways:

- **Reducing anti-apoptotic proteins** – Cancer cells often produce high levels of proteins like **Bcl-2 and Mcl-1**, which act as survival signals. Metformin suppresses these proteins, weakening the cell's defenses against programmed death.
- **Increasing oxidative stress** – While normal cells can tolerate mild fluctuations in energy production, cancer cells are already under extreme metabolic

pressure. Metformin **increases mitochondrial stress**, pushing tumors toward self-destruction.
- **Enhancing chemotherapy-induced apoptosis** – Studies indicate that metformin can make certain chemotherapy drugs **more effective at killing cancer cells**, particularly in breast and prostate cancers.

These findings suggest that metformin not only **slows tumor growth but also actively contributes to the elimination of cancerous cells**, making it a valuable tool in combination treatments.

The Role of p53 in Metformin's Anti-Cancer Effects

Another way metformin influences cancer is by **activating the p53 tumor suppressor gene**, often referred to as the "guardian of the genome." This gene plays a critical role in detecting DNA damage and stopping faulty cells from dividing. In many cancers, p53 is either **mutated or suppressed**, allowing tumors to grow unchecked.

Metformin has been shown to **reactivate p53 in certain cancer cells**, restoring their ability to recognize when something is wrong and initiate self-destruction. This is particularly relevant in aggressive cancers that have found ways to **turn off tumor suppression mechanisms**.

By combining **apoptosis induction, metabolic disruption, and p53 activation**, metformin creates a multi-layered approach to fighting cancer—one that goes beyond traditional treatments and targets cancer's ability to sustain itself at its core. This growing body of evidence is why metformin has become a major focus in **clinical trials** exploring its use as both a **preventative agent and an adjunct cancer therapy**.

Metformin's Impact on the Tumor Microenvironment and Angiogenesis

Cancer is not just a disease of abnormal cell growth—it is a complex system that includes **supporting structures, blood vessels, immune cells, and signaling molecules**, all of which create an environment that helps tumors survive and spread. This is known as the **tumor microenvironment**, and targeting it is a growing area of cancer research.

One of the key ways tumors sustain themselves is by **hijacking the body's blood vessel formation process**, a phenomenon known as **angiogenesis**. By stimulating the growth of new blood vessels, tumors ensure they receive a continuous supply of **oxygen, nutrients, and energy**. This not only allows them to grow beyond their natural size limitations but also provides a pathway for cancer cells to **spread to other organs** through metastasis.

Metformin has been shown to **disrupt angiogenesis**, cutting off the tumor's supply lines and making it harder for cancer to expand. It does this in several ways:

- **Reducing VEGF (vascular endothelial growth factor)** – VEGF is one of the main signals that tells the body to build new blood vessels. Tumors often produce high levels of VEGF to sustain

their growth, but metformin has been shown to **suppress VEGF production**, slowing the formation of new blood vessels.
- **Lowering inflammation in the tumor environment** – Chronic inflammation fuels angiogenesis by keeping tissues in a **constant state of repair and regeneration**. Metformin reduces key inflammatory markers like **TNF-alpha and IL-6**, making the tumor's surroundings less hospitable.
- **Enhancing the effects of anti-angiogenic therapies** – Some cancer drugs, such as bevacizumab (Avastin), work by **blocking blood vessel formation**. Research suggests that metformin may **enhance the effectiveness of these drugs**, improving patient outcomes.

How Metformin Alters the Immune Response Against Cancer

The immune system plays a crucial role in controlling cancer, but tumors have developed ways to **evade immune detection and suppress immune activity**. Some cancers create a highly immunosuppressive environment, making it difficult for the body's natural defenses to attack them.

Metformin appears to **modulate the immune system**, making it more effective at recognizing and destroying cancer cells. Studies have found that metformin:

- **Reprograms immune cells in the tumor microenvironment** – Certain immune cells, like macrophages, can either **attack cancer or help it grow**, depending on their activation state. Metformin has been shown to **shift these cells toward an anti-tumor role**, reducing their support for cancer.
- **Enhances T-cell function** – T-cells are critical for immune-based cancer control, but in some cancers, they become **exhausted** and stop working effectively. Metformin has been shown to **revitalize T-cell function**, making them more aggressive against tumors.
- **Reduces immune-suppressing cells** – Some cancers recruit specialized cells

that **shut down immune responses**. Metformin may help reduce the presence of these cells, restoring the immune system's ability to fight.

By influencing **both angiogenesis and immune suppression**, metformin goes beyond simply slowing cancer growth—it actively **weakens the tumor's defenses**, making it more vulnerable to both natural immune responses and conventional treatments. These discoveries are fueling interest in combining metformin with **immunotherapy**, a field that is rapidly changing the landscape of cancer treatment.

Major Studies Supporting Metformin's Anti-Cancer Properties

The growing interest in metformin as a potential cancer therapy is not based on speculation—**a substantial body of research supports its role in cancer prevention and treatment**. Over the past two decades, multiple large-scale studies, clinical trials, and laboratory experiments have provided compelling evidence that metformin may help **reduce cancer risk, slow tumor progression, and enhance the effectiveness of conventional treatments**.

One of the earliest large-scale studies to highlight metformin's potential came from **retrospective analyses of diabetic patients**. Researchers observed that individuals with type 2 diabetes who took metformin had **significantly lower cancer rates** compared to those taking other diabetes medications. This led to further investigation into metformin's specific effects on different types of cancer.

Key Clinical Studies on Metformin and Cancer

- **The UK Prospective Diabetes Study (UKPDS)** – One of the largest diabetes studies ever conducted, this research revealed that metformin users had a **40% lower risk of developing cancer** compared to those taking insulin or sulfonylureas.

- **JAMA Oncology Breast Cancer Study (2016)** – A clinical trial found that women with early-stage breast cancer who took metformin during treatment had **higher survival rates and lower recurrence** compared to those who did not.
- **Colorectal Cancer and Metformin Study (2020)** – Published in *Cancer Epidemiology*, this study found that patients with colorectal cancer who were on metformin had a **lower risk of disease progression and better response to chemotherapy**.
- **Pancreatic Cancer Survival Study (2015)** – Researchers found that diabetic patients with pancreatic cancer who took metformin lived **significantly longer than those who did not**, suggesting a potential role in slowing this aggressive disease.
- **Meta-Analysis of Multiple Cancers (2018)** – A review of over 50 studies concluded that metformin use was associated with a **significant reduction in cancer incidence and mortality**, particularly in

cancers of the **breast, prostate, lung, and colon**.

How These Findings Are Shaping Future Cancer Treatments

These studies have led to an explosion of interest in metformin's potential role in oncology, with **ongoing clinical trials testing how it can be used alongside chemotherapy, radiation, and immunotherapy**. Researchers are particularly interested in:

- Whether metformin can **prevent cancer recurrence** in survivors who are in remission.
- How metformin **enhances the effectiveness of chemotherapy and radiation**.
- The potential for metformin to be used in **combination with other metabolic therapies**, such as fasting, ketogenic diets, and repurposed drugs like statins and ivermectin.

Although metformin is not yet considered a **first-line cancer treatment**, these findings suggest that it may soon become a **routine**

part of cancer prevention strategies—especially for individuals at **high risk due to metabolic dysfunction, obesity, or insulin resistance**.

With so much promising research, scientists are now working to **refine dosage protocols, determine which cancer types respond best, and explore combination therapies that maximize metformin's effects**. As the next chapters will show, metformin is just one of many repurposed drugs that could change the way cancer is treated in the future.

Chapter 3: Types of Cancer Metformin May Help Prevent and Treat

Metformin and Breast Cancer – Research, Mechanisms, and Clinical Findings

Breast cancer is one of the most well-studied cancers in relation to metformin, with a growing body of evidence suggesting that it may help **reduce risk, slow tumor progression, and improve treatment outcomes**. Given that breast cancer is **highly influenced by metabolic and hormonal factors**, metformin's ability to regulate **insulin, glucose, and inflammation** makes it a strong candidate for both **prevention and adjunct therapy**.

How Metformin Affects Breast Cancer Growth

Breast cancer cells, particularly in **hormone-driven subtypes**, are highly sensitive to insulin and growth factors. Elevated insulin levels act as a **tumor growth signal**, stimulating cell division and creating an environment where cancer thrives. Metformin counters this by:

- **Reducing circulating insulin and IGF-1**, making it harder for tumors to receive excess growth stimulation.
- **Activating AMPK**, which forces cancer cells into an energy-starved state, slowing their growth and making them more vulnerable to treatment.
- **Inhibiting estrogen-driven cancer growth**, which is particularly relevant for **ER-positive breast cancer**, where estrogen fuels tumor expansion.

Beyond these effects, metformin has been shown to **increase the effectiveness of chemotherapy and radiation**, making it a promising addition to standard breast cancer treatment protocols.

Clinical Evidence Supporting Metformin's Role in Breast Cancer

Several major studies have examined metformin's impact on breast cancer, both in terms of **prevention and treatment outcomes**.

- **Women's Health Initiative (WHI) Study (2012)** – This large-scale study found that women with diabetes who were taking metformin had a **lower risk of developing breast cancer** compared to non-users.
- **MA.32 Clinical Trial (2021)** – A randomized trial investigating metformin in early-stage breast cancer patients found that metformin may improve **disease-free survival** in certain breast cancer subtypes.
- **Meta-Analysis of Breast Cancer and Metformin (2018)** – A review of multiple studies concluded that metformin was associated with **reduced breast cancer mortality**, particularly in patients with **high insulin resistance or obesity**.

Researchers are now exploring whether metformin could become a **preventative strategy for high-risk women**, particularly those with **metabolic syndrome, polycystic ovary syndrome (PCOS), or prediabetes**, all of which are associated with **higher breast cancer risk**.

Given its ability to **modify tumor metabolism, enhance standard treatments, and potentially prevent recurrence**, metformin represents an exciting and affordable approach in the fight against breast cancer. Scientists are now expanding their research into other cancers that share similar metabolic vulnerabilities, such as **colorectal cancer**, which will be explored in the next section.

Metformin and Colorectal Cancer – Gut Health, Microbiome Impact, and Tumor Prevention

Colorectal cancer is one of the most metabolically influenced cancers, making it an important area of study for **metformin's potential protective effects**. Research suggests that metformin may not only **lower the risk of developing colorectal cancer** but also **improve outcomes for those already diagnosed**. Given its ability to **regulate insulin, influence gut microbiota, and reduce inflammation**, metformin is emerging as a powerful tool in colorectal cancer prevention and therapy.

How Metformin Influences Colorectal Cancer Growth

Colorectal cancer development is closely linked to **metabolic dysfunction, chronic inflammation, and an imbalanced gut microbiome**. Insulin resistance and high blood sugar have been associated with increased tumor formation in the colon, as excess glucose provides fuel for abnormal cell growth.

Metformin helps disrupt these cancer-promoting conditions by:

- **Lowering insulin and glucose levels**, reducing the energy supply that colorectal tumors thrive on.
- **Activating AMPK**, which slows down cancer cell proliferation and enhances cellular repair mechanisms.
- **Reducing inflammation in the gut**, particularly by lowering pro-inflammatory markers such as **TNF-**

alpha and IL-6, which have been linked to colorectal tumor progression.

One of the most fascinating areas of research on metformin and colorectal cancer is its **impact on gut microbiota**. Studies suggest that metformin **promotes beneficial gut bacteria** while inhibiting harmful microbes that contribute to chronic inflammation. This shift in microbiome composition may play a **direct role in lowering colorectal cancer risk**, as an unhealthy gut environment is a major factor in tumor development.

Clinical Evidence Supporting Metformin's Role in Colorectal Cancer

Several population-based studies and clinical trials have found **a significant association between metformin use and reduced colorectal cancer incidence**.

- **Meta-Analysis of 17 Studies (2016)** – This large-scale review found that metformin users had a **27% lower risk of developing colorectal cancer** compared to non-users.

- **Colorectal Cancer Survival Study (2020)** – Patients with colorectal cancer who were taking metformin showed **improved survival rates and better responses to chemotherapy**.
- **Gut Microbiome and Metformin Study (2021)** – Research showed that metformin positively influenced gut bacteria, increasing species linked to **reduced inflammation and improved gut barrier function**.

Given the close connection between **diet, gut health, and colorectal cancer**, metformin may be particularly beneficial when combined with other metabolic interventions such as **a fiber-rich diet, fasting strategies, and probiotics**.

With colorectal cancer rates rising—particularly in younger individuals—researchers are now looking at whether **metformin should be used preventatively in high-risk groups**, such as those with **obesity, type 2 diabetes, inflammatory bowel disease (IBD), or a strong family history of colorectal cancer**.

As scientists continue to explore metformin's role in digestive health, another area of growing interest is **prostate cancer**, which shares similar metabolic vulnerabilities and may also respond well to metformin-based interventions.

Metformin and Prostate Cancer – Insulin Resistance, Testosterone Regulation, and Clinical Findings

Prostate cancer is one of the most common cancers in men, and like other hormone-driven cancers, it appears to be **strongly influenced by metabolism and insulin resistance**. Research suggests that **elevated blood sugar, chronic inflammation, and high insulin levels** create an environment where prostate cancer can develop and progress more aggressively. This makes metformin an intriguing candidate for both **reducing prostate cancer risk and improving outcomes in diagnosed patients**.

How Metformin May Help Fight Prostate Cancer

Prostate cancer cells have been shown to **overexpress insulin receptors**, meaning they are highly responsive to **elevated insulin and IGF-1 (insulin-like growth factor-1)**. When insulin and IGF-1 levels are high, they provide **constant growth stimulation to prostate cancer cells**, allowing tumors to grow more aggressively.

Metformin helps counteract this process by:

- **Lowering insulin and IGF-1 levels**, which reduces the excessive growth signals that prostate cancer relies on.
- **Suppressing inflammation**, particularly by reducing cytokines like **IL-6**, which has been linked to prostate cancer progression.
- **Inhibiting mTOR**, a pathway that drives uncontrolled cell proliferation in aggressive prostate cancers.

Beyond insulin regulation, metformin has also been studied for its role in **testosterone metabolism**, another key factor in prostate cancer development. While metformin does not directly lower testosterone levels, it

improves hormone balance by reducing insulin resistance, which in turn **modifies androgen signaling in ways that may slow tumor growth**.

Clinical Studies on Metformin and Prostate Cancer

Several major studies have examined the effects of metformin on **prostate cancer risk, progression, and treatment response**:

- **Canadian Prostate Cancer Study (2014)** – Found that men taking metformin had a **reduced risk of developing advanced prostate cancer** compared to non-users.
- **Metformin and Prostate Cancer Recurrence Study (2019)** – A trial examining post-surgery patients found that metformin use was linked to **a lower risk of cancer recurrence** following prostate removal.
- **Metformin and Androgen Deprivation Therapy (2021)** – Research suggested that metformin may **enhance the effectiveness of hormonal therapies** like androgen deprivation therapy

(ADT), which is commonly used to slow prostate cancer growth.

Given that prostate cancer is often **slow-growing**, some researchers are now investigating whether metformin could be used in a **"watchful waiting" approach**, where men with early-stage prostate cancer take metformin to **help slow tumor progression without immediately resorting to aggressive treatments**.

The connection between **prostate cancer, metabolic health, and inflammation** is still being explored, but the findings so far suggest that **metformin could serve as an accessible and effective intervention for both prevention and long-term management**.

As scientists continue to study metformin's effects on hormone-driven cancers, another area of interest is **pancreatic cancer**—a far more aggressive disease where metabolic interventions may offer much-needed treatment advances.

Metformin and Pancreatic Cancer – Targeting Metabolic Pathways in an Aggressive Disease

Pancreatic cancer is one of the most **aggressive and deadly cancers**, with a notoriously poor survival rate. Unlike some slower-growing cancers, pancreatic cancer is **highly resistant to treatment** and often diagnosed at an advanced stage, leaving few effective options. Given the urgent need for better therapies, researchers have turned their attention to metformin, which has shown **promising effects in slowing tumor progression and improving survival in some pancreatic cancer patients**.

How Pancreatic Cancer Exploits Metabolism to Grow

Pancreatic cancer is deeply connected to **metabolic dysfunction**, with insulin resistance, chronic inflammation, and obesity being major risk factors. Many pancreatic tumors **overexpress insulin and glucose transporters**, making them highly dependent on sugar and insulin signaling for rapid growth. This is why **people with type 2 diabetes have a significantly higher risk of developing pancreatic cancer**, and why controlling blood sugar and insulin levels is considered a key strategy in prevention.

Metformin disrupts this process by:

- **Lowering insulin and IGF-1**, cutting off key growth signals that pancreatic tumors depend on.
- **Activating AMPK**, which shifts cancer cells into a metabolic state where they struggle to generate the energy needed for rapid division.
- **Inhibiting the mTOR pathway**, a major driver of pancreatic tumor growth and resistance to treatment.
- **Reducing inflammation**, particularly by suppressing cytokines and oxidative stress that contribute to cancer progression.

Pancreatic cancer cells are known for their ability to **quickly adapt to chemotherapy and develop resistance**, making them difficult to eliminate. However, metformin's **metabolic-disrupting effects** appear to weaken cancer cells, making them **more vulnerable to chemotherapy and radiation treatments**.

Clinical Studies on Metformin and Pancreatic Cancer

While pancreatic cancer is notoriously difficult to treat, multiple studies have suggested that metformin may provide **a survival advantage, particularly in diabetic patients**:

- **Mayo Clinic Pancreatic Cancer Study (2015)** – Found that diabetic patients taking metformin had **a longer median survival time** than those not on metformin.
- **Metformin and Chemotherapy Synergy Study (2017)** – Research showed that metformin enhanced the effects of **gemcitabine**, a common chemotherapy drug used in pancreatic cancer treatment.
- **Meta-Analysis of Metformin in Pancreatic Cancer (2020)** – A review

of multiple studies found that metformin use was associated with a **small but significant improvement in overall survival**, particularly in early-stage patients.

Despite these promising findings, pancreatic cancer remains a **highly aggressive disease**, and metformin alone is not a cure. However, researchers are now testing **combination therapies**, exploring whether metformin can **work alongside fasting protocols, ketogenic diets, and other metabolic interventions** to further **weaken tumors and improve treatment response**.

Because pancreatic cancer has such strong ties to **metabolic dysfunction**, understanding the role of metformin in both **prevention and treatment** may offer new strategies to fight this devastating disease. As research expands, scientists are also looking at how metformin might influence **other difficult-to-treat cancers, including lung cancer and rare malignancies**.

Metformin and Lung Cancer – A New Avenue in Treatment and Prevention

Lung cancer remains one of the **leading causes of cancer-related deaths worldwide**, with survival rates heavily dependent on early detection and treatment response. While traditionally linked to smoking, a growing body of research suggests that **metabolic factors also play a role in lung cancer progression**, making metformin an interesting candidate for both **prevention and adjunct therapy**.

How Metformin May Impact Lung Cancer Progression

Lung cancer cells, particularly in non-small cell lung cancer (NSCLC), rely on **elevated glucose metabolism and insulin signaling** to sustain their aggressive growth. Many lung tumors also **overexpress mTOR and IGF-1 pathways**, both of which promote rapid cell division and resistance to treatment.

Metformin's effects on lung cancer may include:

- **Lowering insulin and glucose availability**, depriving tumors of essential fuel.
- **Suppressing mTOR**, a pathway that accelerates tumor cell growth.
- **Enhancing the effects of radiation and chemotherapy**, making standard treatments more effective.
- **Reducing inflammation in the lungs**, which is a known contributor to lung cancer development, especially in non-smokers.

Beyond these metabolic effects, metformin has been studied for its ability to **increase sensitivity to immune-based treatments**, such as checkpoint inhibitors, which have become a breakthrough in lung cancer care.

Clinical Evidence Supporting Metformin's Role in Lung Cancer

While more research is needed, several studies have found that metformin may offer **both protective and therapeutic benefits** for lung cancer patients:

- **MD Anderson Cancer Center Study (2014)** – Found that diabetic patients

taking metformin had a **significantly lower risk of developing lung cancer** compared to those on other diabetes medications.
- **Metformin and Radiation Therapy Study (2016)** – Research indicated that metformin improved **tumor response to radiation therapy**, leading to better survival outcomes.
- **Lung Cancer and Immunotherapy Study (2021)** – Showed that metformin may **enhance the effectiveness of immune checkpoint inhibitors**, a class of drugs that help the immune system attack cancer cells.

These findings suggest that **metformin's metabolic-disrupting effects extend beyond traditional metabolic cancers like breast and colorectal cancer**, influencing even highly aggressive cancers like **lung cancer**.

Future Directions in Metformin and Lung Cancer Research

Scientists are now investigating how metformin could be combined with **fasting**

protocols, ketogenic diets, and additional repurposed drugs to enhance lung cancer treatment. Since lung cancer often develops **resistance to chemotherapy and radiation**, the ability to **weaken tumor metabolism through non-toxic, low-cost interventions** could significantly improve patient outcomes.

With its ability to influence **glucose metabolism, tumor growth pathways, and immune response**, metformin stands as an **exciting prospect in lung cancer research**, paving the way for new, **less toxic treatment strategies** that complement existing therapies.

As research continues, metformin's role in **rare and aggressive cancers** is also being explored, offering further potential for **repurposed drug therapies in oncology**.

Chapter 4: Low-Dose Naltrexone (LDN) and Immunomodulation

How LDN Influences the Immune System and Its Potential Role in Cancer Therapy

Low-dose naltrexone (LDN) is one of the most intriguing **repurposed drugs** being explored for cancer treatment. Originally developed to **block opioid receptors and treat addiction**, naltrexone was later discovered to have **profound effects on immune regulation** when taken in very low doses. This discovery has led to increasing interest in LDN as a potential **cancer therapy**, particularly for its ability to **enhance immune function, reduce inflammation, and improve overall cellular resilience**.

At its core, LDN works by **modulating the body's opioid receptors**, which are not just involved in pain management but also play a significant role in **immune system function and cellular repair**. When taken in low doses, LDN **briefly blocks opioid receptors**, triggering a **rebound effect** that leads to

increased endorphin production. This has been shown to have wide-ranging benefits, including:

- **Boosting immune system activity**, making it easier for the body to detect and attack cancer cells.
- **Reducing chronic inflammation**, a major driver of cancer progression.
- **Regulating abnormal cell growth**, helping prevent uncontrolled division.

What makes LDN particularly promising is its ability to **target cancer's ability to evade immune detection**. Many cancers create an **immunosuppressive environment**, shutting down the body's natural defense mechanisms. LDN appears to **counteract this effect**, potentially making tumors more vulnerable to attack by the immune system.

LDN and Cancer Immunotherapy – A Synergistic Approach

LDN is now being explored as a **complementary treatment alongside immunotherapy**, one of the most exciting developments in modern cancer care.

Immunotherapy drugs, such as **checkpoint inhibitors**, work by removing the "brakes" on the immune system, allowing it to aggressively fight tumors. However, **not all patients respond to immunotherapy**, leading researchers to investigate whether LDN could **enhance immune responsiveness** in those who otherwise show resistance.

In addition to its direct effects on the immune system, LDN may also play a role in **regulating inflammation-driven cancers**, particularly those that thrive in a chronic inflammatory state. These include:

- **Breast cancer**
- **Ovarian cancer**
- **Pancreatic cancer**

As research continues, LDN is emerging as a **low-cost, low-risk adjunct therapy** that may help reshape the way we think about cancer treatment, focusing not just on destroying tumors, but on **optimizing the body's own ability to fight back**.

The Connection Between Endorphins, Inflammation, and Cancer Cell Control

One of the most fascinating aspects of **low-dose naltrexone (LDN)** is its ability to **increase endorphin levels**, which has significant implications for **immune function, inflammation regulation, and cancer growth suppression**. Endorphins, commonly known as the body's natural painkillers, do far more than just improve mood—they play a critical role in **cell growth regulation and immune surveillance**, both of which are key factors in cancer progression.

Research has shown that **many cancer patients have abnormally low endorphin levels**, which may contribute to their **weakened immune response and increased tumor growth**. Since LDN works by temporarily blocking opioid receptors, it creates a **rebound effect**, prompting the body to produce more endorphins. This increase in endorphins appears to have several cancer-fighting effects:

- **Strengthening the immune response** – Endorphins help stimulate **natural killer (NK) cells and T-cells**, which are essential for detecting and destroying cancer cells before they multiply.
- **Regulating cell growth** – Cancer cells bypass normal growth control mechanisms, but endorphins help **restore balance** by promoting apoptosis (programmed cell death) in abnormal cells.
- **Reducing inflammation** – Chronic inflammation is a key driver of many cancers, and endorphins have been shown to suppress inflammatory pathways, particularly **TNF-alpha and IL-6**, both of which are linked to tumor growth.

How Chronic Inflammation Fuels Cancer—and How LDN May Help

Many cancers thrive in **highly inflamed environments**, where inflammatory molecules act as **fertilizer for tumor growth**. Inflammation promotes:

- **Increased blood vessel formation (angiogenesis)**, allowing tumors to access more oxygen and nutrients.
- **Suppression of immune surveillance**, making it easier for cancer cells to evade detection.
- **Damage to healthy tissues**, creating an environment where cancer cells can spread more easily.

LDN appears to **interrupt this cycle**, helping to turn off the constant inflammatory signaling that allows cancer to grow unchecked. This is particularly relevant for cancers that are strongly linked to **chronic inflammation, such as breast, ovarian, colorectal, and pancreatic cancer**.

By **modulating immune activity, restoring endorphin levels, and reducing inflammation**, LDN offers a **multi-pronged approach** to cancer control. Its ability to **enhance the effects of conventional treatments, support immune function, and improve overall well-being** is what makes it an increasingly valuable tool in cancer therapy research.

Research on LDN in Breast, Ovarian, and Pancreatic Cancers

The potential of **low-dose naltrexone (LDN) in cancer therapy** is gaining traction, particularly in cancers driven by **immune suppression and chronic inflammation**. While LDN is not yet a mainstream cancer treatment, early studies and clinical observations suggest that it may play a role in **slowing tumor growth, enhancing immune response, and improving treatment outcomes** in several aggressive cancer types, including **breast, ovarian, and pancreatic cancers**.

LDN and Breast Cancer

Breast cancer is strongly influenced by **hormonal imbalances, inflammation, and immune system dysfunction**. Many breast tumors use immune suppression as a strategy to evade detection, making it harder for the body to fight back. LDN appears to help by:

- **Increasing natural killer (NK) cell activity**, improving the body's ability to recognize and attack cancerous cells.
- **Reducing inflammatory cytokines**, which are known to fuel breast tumor progression, particularly in estrogen receptor-positive (ER+) cancers.
- **Enhancing chemotherapy effectiveness**, potentially making conventional treatments more successful.

A **2017 study published in *Cancer Immunology Research* suggested that LDN may help improve immune function in breast cancer patients** who are undergoing standard treatments, possibly reducing recurrence rates.

LDN and Ovarian Cancer

Ovarian cancer remains one of the most **challenging cancers to detect and treat**, largely because it often spreads before symptoms appear. Like breast cancer, ovarian cancer is influenced by **immune evasion and inflammation**, and some researchers believe LDN may help improve patient outcomes.

In preliminary studies, LDN has shown promise in:

- **Reducing tumor-associated inflammation**, which is a major factor in ovarian cancer progression.
- **Boosting endorphin levels**, which may help regulate tumor growth and improve immune function.
- **Enhancing response to chemotherapy**, particularly in **platinum-resistant ovarian cancer**, a form of the disease that does not respond well to conventional treatments.

While large-scale clinical trials are still needed, early case reports suggest that LDN **may help slow progression and improve quality of life in ovarian cancer patients**.

LDN and Pancreatic Cancer

Pancreatic cancer is one of the most **aggressive and deadly cancers**, with a low survival rate due to its rapid spread and resistance to treatment. Given its strong links to **chronic inflammation and immune suppression**, researchers have explored whether LDN's **immunomodulatory effects** could be beneficial.

LDN may help pancreatic cancer patients by:

- **Reducing tumor-promoting inflammation**, particularly by lowering cytokines like **TNF-alpha and IL-6**.
- **Enhancing immune system activation**, improving the body's ability to attack cancer cells.
- **Potentially increasing sensitivity to chemotherapy**, making standard treatments more effective.

A **small clinical case study in 2016** documented a pancreatic cancer patient who incorporated LDN alongside conventional therapies and experienced **longer-than-expected survival and reduced tumor growth**. While anecdotal, findings like this have encouraged further research.

What the Future Holds for LDN in Cancer Treatment

Although LDN is not yet a widely accepted cancer treatment, the **early research and**

clinical reports suggest significant promise. As more oncologists explore **the role of immune system modulation in cancer treatment**, LDN may become a **low-cost, low-risk adjunct therapy** used to enhance conventional approaches.

Current and future trials will focus on:

- How LDN interacts with **chemotherapy and immunotherapy**.
- Whether it **reduces recurrence rates** in cancer survivors.
- Its impact on **long-term survival in inflammatory-driven cancers**.

For now, LDN remains **an experimental but highly promising option**, one that is drawing increasing interest as a potential tool in **the broader landscape of repurposed drugs for cancer therapy**.

How to Use LDN – Dosing Strategies and Safety Considerations

Low-dose naltrexone (LDN) is distinct from the standard high-dose naltrexone used for opioid addiction. In cancer therapy, LDN is typically taken in **microdoses ranging from 1.5 mg to 4.5 mg per day**, which appears to be the optimal range for its **immune-enhancing and anti-inflammatory effects**.

Unlike conventional cancer drugs, LDN does not attack cancer cells directly. Instead, it works by **modulating immune function, increasing endorphin levels, and reducing inflammation**—all of which contribute to a less favorable environment for cancer growth. This makes LDN a valuable **adjunct therapy**, rather than a standalone treatment.

Dosing Protocol for LDN in Cancer Therapy

Since LDN works by temporarily blocking opioid receptors, it's typically taken **once daily, before bedtime**. This allows the body to **experience a rebound effect in endorphin production** during the night, which has been linked to its beneficial effects on immune system regulation.

The most common **dosing approach** involves:

- **Starting with 1.5 mg per day** to assess tolerance.
- **Gradually increasing the dose** every 7–10 days, reaching **3.0 mg, then 4.5 mg per day**, if well tolerated.
- **Maintaining a stable dose** at **3.0–4.5 mg per day**, depending on individual response.

Because LDN influences immune function, some patients **report mild symptoms when first starting**, including **temporary sleep disturbances, vivid dreams, or mild headaches**. These effects are usually short-lived and **resolve as the body adjusts**.

Who Should Be Cautious When Using LDN?

LDN is generally **well tolerated and has minimal side effects**, especially when compared to traditional cancer treatments. However, certain individuals should consult with a healthcare provider before using LDN, particularly those who:

- Are taking **opioid-based pain medications**, as LDN can interfere with their effects.
- Have undergone **recent organ transplants**, as it may alter immune function.
- Have autoimmune conditions, as responses to LDN can be **variable**.

Because LDN is **not an FDA-approved cancer treatment**, it is often **prescribed off-label**. However, given its **low risk and emerging clinical interest**, many integrative oncologists are beginning to incorporate it into treatment plans, particularly in patients with **hormone-driven and inflammation-related cancers**.

How Long Should LDN Be Used in Cancer Therapy?

Since LDN works **by improving immune function over time**, most patients take it for an **extended period**, often **months to years**. Some research suggests that continuing LDN after conventional treatment **may reduce the risk of cancer recurrence**, though more studies are needed to confirm this effect.

As researchers continue to explore **how LDN interacts with chemotherapy, immunotherapy, and metabolic treatments**, its role in cancer care **is likely to expand**, making it a promising tool in **repurposed drug therapy** for cancer.

Combining LDN with Other Therapies for Enhanced Immune Response

Low-dose naltrexone (LDN) is most effective when used as part of a **multi-pronged approach to cancer treatment**, rather than as a standalone therapy. Because LDN primarily **modulates the immune system and reduces inflammation**, it complements several other repurposed drugs and metabolic therapies that **target cancer through different mechanisms**.

By combining LDN with other interventions that promote **immune function, metabolic regulation, and inflammation control**, patients may achieve a **synergistic effect** that enhances treatment outcomes and improves quality of life.

LDN and Metformin – A Dual Approach to Cancer Metabolism and Immunity

Metformin and LDN are often discussed together because they target **two of cancer's biggest survival mechanisms: metabolic dysfunction and immune evasion**.

- **Metformin reduces insulin and IGF-1 levels**, starving tumors of their primary energy sources.
- **LDN enhances immune surveillance**, making it harder for cancer cells to escape detection.
- **Both drugs reduce inflammation**, lowering cytokines such as **IL-6 and TNF-alpha**, which fuel tumor progression.

This combination is particularly promising for **hormone-driven cancers like breast and ovarian cancer**, where **both metabolic and immune factors** contribute to disease progression.

LDN and Ivermectin – Targeting Cancer's Survival Pathways

Ivermectin, another **repurposed drug with emerging anti-cancer potential**, has been studied for its ability to **disrupt cancer cell signaling and enhance immune response**. When paired with LDN, the effects may be even stronger:

- **Ivermectin blocks WNT signaling**, a pathway that some cancers use to resist treatment.
- **LDN boosts T-cell and natural killer (NK) cell activity**, improving immune function.
- **Both drugs suppress inflammation and oxidative stress**, making it harder for cancer to thrive.

While research is still early, some oncologists are beginning to explore whether this combination **could be useful in cancers with immune suppression, such as lung, pancreatic, and colorectal cancers**.

LDN with Fasting and Ketogenic Diets – Supporting Metabolic Health

Since LDN works **best in an anti-inflammatory environment**, combining it with **intermittent fasting or a ketogenic diet** may further enhance its effects. These dietary strategies help:

- **Lower blood sugar and insulin**, making it harder for cancer to grow.
- **Reduce systemic inflammation**, which complements LDN's immune-modulating properties.
- **Improve mitochondrial function**, making cancer cells more vulnerable to treatment.

Some studies suggest that fasting may also **increase the effectiveness of chemotherapy and immunotherapy**, meaning that using LDN in combination with fasting protocols **could provide an extra layer of protection**.

LDN as Part of a Comprehensive Cancer Treatment Strategy

Because LDN is a **low-risk, low-cost therapy**, it has become an **appealing option** for those looking to complement conventional treatments or **reduce recurrence risk after remission**. When used alongside other repurposed drugs, dietary interventions, and standard cancer therapies, it may help:

- **Enhance overall immune response**.
- **Reduce the risk of treatment resistance**.
- **Improve long-term outcomes**.

While LDN alone is not a cure, its ability to **fine-tune immune function, lower inflammation, and improve response to other therapies** makes it one of the most promising **adjunct treatments** in the growing field of **repurposed drugs for cancer**.

Chapter 5: Statins, Antibiotics, and Blood Thinners – Surprising Anti-Cancer Agents

How Statins May Reduce Cancer Risk and Slow Tumor Growth

Statins, best known for their role in **lowering cholesterol**, have unexpectedly emerged as **potential cancer-fighting drugs**. Originally designed to block the liver's production of cholesterol, statins also interfere with critical **cell growth and signaling pathways** that cancer cells rely on to multiply.

Research suggests that statins may help slow tumor progression by:

- **Disrupting the mevalonate pathway**, which cancer cells use to produce vital growth-promoting compounds.
- **Inhibiting cell proliferation**, making it harder for tumors to expand.
- **Inducing apoptosis (programmed cell death)**, forcing cancer cells to self-destruct.
- **Reducing inflammation**, which is a major driver of many cancers.

Several large population studies have found that people taking statins for cholesterol control **may have a lower risk of developing certain cancers**, particularly **breast, prostate, colorectal, and lung cancer**.

Statins and Chemotherapy – A Potentially Powerful Combination

Beyond their preventative effects, statins have been shown to **enhance the effectiveness of chemotherapy** in some cancers. By weakening cancer cells and making them more vulnerable to attack, statins may:

- **Increase tumor sensitivity to chemotherapy drugs** such as **doxorubicin and paclitaxel**.
- **Reduce the ability of cancer cells to repair DNA damage**, making treatments more effective.
- **Limit the spread of cancer by disrupting tumor cell migration**.

A **2019 study published in *Cancer Research*** found that **statins improved survival rates**

in breast cancer patients when used alongside standard chemotherapy.

Which Cancers May Respond Best to Statin Therapy?

While statins are not yet a standard cancer treatment, they are being actively researched for their effects on:

- **Breast cancer** – By reducing cholesterol-derived estrogen production, statins may slow hormone-driven tumor growth.
- **Prostate cancer** – Statin users have been observed to have **lower recurrence rates** after prostate cancer treatment.
- **Colorectal cancer** – Statins interfere with tumor-promoting inflammation in the gut.
- **Lung cancer** – Some studies suggest statins may reduce the likelihood of lung cancer spreading to other organs.

Because statins are **low-cost and widely available**, they represent a **promising addition to cancer prevention strategies**, particularly for those at **high risk due to**

metabolic syndrome, obesity, or chronic inflammation.

With ongoing trials exploring **optimal dosing, treatment timing, and combination therapies**, statins may soon become an important part of **repurposed drug protocols for cancer care**.

The Role of Doxycycline and Other Antibiotics in Targeting Cancer Stem Cells

Antibiotics are traditionally used to **fight bacterial infections**, but some of them—particularly doxycycline—have shown unexpected **anti-cancer effects**, specifically in targeting **cancer stem cells**. Cancer stem cells (CSCs) are a **major reason for tumor recurrence and treatment resistance**, as they can survive chemotherapy and regenerate new cancer cells. Finding a way to weaken or eliminate CSCs is a critical goal in cancer therapy, and **doxycycline may play a key role** in this process.

How Doxycycline Affects Cancer Stem Cells

Unlike normal cancer cells, CSCs rely on **mitochondrial energy production** rather than the glycolysis-heavy metabolism seen in many tumors. Doxycycline interferes with **mitochondrial protein synthesis**, disrupting the energy supply CSCs need to survive. This effect has been shown to:

- **Reduce CSC populations in tumors**, making them more susceptible to treatment.
- **Prevent chemotherapy resistance**, as CSCs are often the reason cancers return after treatment.
- **Inhibit tumor regrowth**, potentially lowering recurrence rates.

A **2015 study in *Oncotarget*** found that **doxycycline significantly reduced CSC numbers in breast, lung, and prostate cancer models**, leading to greater treatment success when combined with chemotherapy.

Other Antibiotics with Anti-Cancer Properties

Beyond doxycycline, several other antibiotics have been studied for their ability to **weaken tumors and disrupt cancer metabolism**:

- **Azithromycin and erythromycin** – These antibiotics also target **mitochondrial function**, weakening cancer cells.
- **Clarithromycin** – Often used in stomach ulcer treatments, clarithromycin has shown potential in **reducing tumor-promoting inflammation**.
- **Rifampicin** – Some studies suggest it may interfere with **cancer cell signaling and immune evasion mechanisms**.

Because antibiotics like doxycycline are already **widely available and inexpensive**, they represent a **practical and low-risk option** for integration into cancer treatment protocols.

Combining Antibiotics with Other Cancer Therapies

Early research suggests that antibiotics may work best when **combined with other repurposed drugs and metabolic therapies**, such as:

- **Doxycycline + Metformin** – While doxycycline targets cancer stem cells, metformin weakens tumor metabolism, creating a **dual-attack strategy**.
- **Doxycycline + Fasting or Ketogenic Diets** – Since fasting and ketogenic diets reduce glucose availability, they may **enhance the effects of doxycycline by starving cancer cells further**.
- **Doxycycline + Chemotherapy** – By making cancer stem cells more vulnerable, doxycycline may **increase the effectiveness of standard cancer treatments**.

Although antibiotics alone are **not a cure for cancer**, their ability to **target cancer stem cells and disrupt mitochondrial function** makes them an exciting area of **drug repurposing research**. Future clinical trials will determine whether antibiotics like doxycycline **can become part of standard cancer therapy**, particularly for aggressive and treatment-resistant tumors.

How Blood Thinners Like Dipyridamole May Inhibit Tumor Angiogenesis

Blood thinners, or **anticoagulants**, are primarily used to **prevent blood clots** in conditions like heart disease and stroke. However, research has revealed that certain blood thinners, particularly **dipyridamole**, may have unexpected **anti-cancer effects** by interfering with **tumor angiogenesis**—the process by which cancer cells stimulate the formation of new blood vessels to fuel their growth.

Tumors require a **constant supply of oxygen and nutrients**, and they accomplish this by hijacking the body's natural ability to **grow new blood vessels (angiogenesis)**. The faster a tumor can establish its own blood supply, the more aggressively it can grow and spread. Many modern cancer treatments, such as **bevacizumab (Avastin)**, work by **blocking angiogenesis**. Interestingly, some widely available blood thinners appear to have **a similar effect**.

How Dipyridamole May Disrupt Tumor Growth

Dipyridamole is a **platelet aggregation inhibitor**, meaning it prevents blood cells from sticking together and forming clots. But beyond its role in cardiovascular health, it has been shown to:

- **Reduce tumor-induced blood vessel formation**, limiting the supply of nutrients to cancer cells.
- **Disrupt platelet-tumor interactions**, which can help prevent metastasis.
- **Enhance chemotherapy delivery**, as improved blood flow allows more **anti-cancer drugs to reach tumors**.

A **2019 study published in *Cancer Medicine*** found that **dipyridamole inhibited tumor growth in colorectal and breast cancer models**, supporting the idea that it may have applications in **cancer treatment and prevention**.

Other Blood Thinners with Potential Anti-Cancer Effects

Besides dipyridamole, several other anticoagulants have been explored for their **cancer-fighting potential**:

- **Heparin** – Shown to **reduce metastasis** in some cancers by preventing tumor cells from using platelets as a shield.
- **Warfarin** – Some studies suggest that warfarin **lowers cancer incidence**, possibly due to its effects on tumor blood supply.
- **Low-molecular-weight heparin (LMWH)** – Used in some cancer patients to reduce clotting risk, LMWH has also demonstrated **anti-angiogenic effects**.

While blood thinners are not currently considered **first-line cancer treatments**, their ability to **reduce angiogenesis and prevent metastasis** has led researchers to explore whether they could be used alongside standard therapies.

Who May Benefit from Blood Thinners in Cancer Therapy?

Certain groups of cancer patients may benefit the most from **anticoagulant therapy**, particularly those at **high risk of blood clots**, which can be a serious complication of both cancer and chemotherapy. Some researchers are investigating whether **using blood thinners early in cancer treatment** could help slow tumor progression and improve survival rates.

As with any repurposed drug, the key challenge is **finding the right balance between benefits and risks**. Since blood thinners can increase **bleeding risks**, they are not suitable for all cancer patients. However, for those with **metastatic disease, aggressive tumor growth, or clotting complications**, they may offer **an additional layer of protection against cancer progression**.

Ongoing clinical trials are exploring how **anticoagulants like dipyridamole can be combined with other cancer therapies**, particularly **angiogenesis inhibitors, chemotherapy, and metabolic treatments**. If successful, blood thinners could become another **low-cost, widely available tool** in the fight against cancer.

How These Drugs Can Be Used Together or with Standard Cancer Treatments

While **statins, antibiotics, and blood thinners** each have distinct mechanisms of action, they all share a **common ability to weaken cancer's survival strategies**. By **disrupting tumor metabolism, inflammation, and blood supply**, these drugs have the potential to **enhance standard cancer treatments**, including chemotherapy, radiation, and immunotherapy.

Using **multiple repurposed drugs in combination** is a growing area of cancer research. Rather than relying on a **single therapy**, a combination approach aims to **target cancer from multiple angles at once**, reducing its ability to adapt and resist treatment.

Synergistic Drug Combinations for Cancer Treatment

Certain combinations of repurposed drugs have shown promise in **clinical and preclinical studies**, particularly when used alongside standard treatments.

- **Statins + Chemotherapy** – Statins have been found to **increase cancer cell sensitivity to chemotherapy**, particularly in **breast, prostate, and colorectal cancers**. By inhibiting the mevalonate pathway, statins reduce cancer cells' ability to **repair DNA damage caused by chemotherapy drugs**.
- **Doxycycline + Metformin** – Doxycycline targets **cancer stem cells**, while metformin **disrupts cancer's energy metabolism**. This combination may **reduce the likelihood of recurrence** by eliminating both **cancerous cells and their resistant stem cell populations**.
- **Blood Thinners + Angiogenesis Inhibitors** – Since blood thinners like **dipyridamole** and **heparin** reduce **tumor blood supply**, they may work synergistically with **anti-angiogenic cancer drugs like bevacizumab (Avastin)**.

In addition to these drug combinations, **dietary and metabolic strategies**—such as **fasting, ketogenic diets, and intermittent**

calorie restriction—are being explored to further **enhance the effectiveness of these therapies**.

Can These Drugs Be Used for Cancer Prevention?

Beyond their potential in active cancer treatment, some of these repurposed drugs may also be useful in **cancer prevention**, particularly for **high-risk individuals**.

- **Statins and metformin** have both been linked to **lower cancer risk** in long-term population studies, particularly in individuals with **obesity, diabetes, or metabolic syndrome**.
- **Low-dose aspirin or blood thinners** may help **prevent metastasis** by limiting tumor blood vessel formation.
- **Doxycycline and other antibiotics** could play a role in **reducing chronic inflammation** that contributes to cancer initiation.

While more research is needed, these findings suggest that **repurposed drugs could become an affordable and widely**

accessible tool for reducing both **cancer risk and recurrence rates** in the future.

Next Steps in Research and Clinical Use

With growing interest in **drug repurposing**, several clinical trials are underway to determine the **most effective ways to integrate these drugs into cancer treatment**. Researchers are particularly interested in:

- **Identifying which cancers respond best to these treatments**.
- **Determining optimal dosing strategies** to balance effectiveness and safety.
- **Understanding how these drugs interact with each other and with standard cancer therapies**.

While these repurposed drugs are **not a replacement for conventional treatments**, their ability to **enhance therapy, reduce recurrence risk, and improve survival outcomes** makes them an exciting area of cancer research. As studies continue, oncologists and patients alike may soon have a new set of tools to fight cancer more effectively.

Safety Concerns and Monitoring When Using These Drugs for Cancer Therapy

While **repurposed drugs** such as statins, antibiotics, and blood thinners show promise in cancer treatment, they must be used **cautiously and under medical supervision**. Each of these drugs has **potential side effects, interactions, and contraindications**, which means that careful dosing and monitoring are essential.

Potential Risks and Side Effects

- **Statins** – Although generally well tolerated, statins may cause **muscle pain, liver enzyme elevations, and metabolic changes**. In rare cases, they have been linked to **rhabdomyolysis**, a serious condition involving muscle breakdown. Patients with **pre-existing liver disease or severe metabolic disorders** may need closer monitoring.

- **Doxycycline and Other Antibiotics** – Long-term antibiotic use can **disrupt gut microbiota**, leading to digestive issues or increased susceptibility to infections. Some antibiotics may also **increase sensitivity to sunlight or interact with chemotherapy drugs**.
- **Blood Thinners (Dipyridamole, Heparin, Warfarin, etc.)** – The main risk of anticoagulants is **bleeding**, particularly in patients undergoing surgery or those with blood clotting disorders. Combining blood thinners with chemotherapy or radiation may require **frequent monitoring of clotting factors**.

Understanding these risks is crucial for integrating repurposed drugs safely into a cancer treatment plan.

Who Should Be Monitored Closely?

Certain individuals may need **regular check-ups and blood tests** to ensure these medications are working as intended without causing harm. This includes:

- **Patients on multiple cancer therapies** – Some chemotherapy and immunotherapy drugs interact with repurposed drugs, potentially enhancing or reducing their effects.
- **Individuals with liver or kidney disease** – Since many of these drugs are **processed by the liver or excreted through the kidneys**, patients with impaired organ function may require **dose adjustments**.
- **Those at risk for bleeding disorders** – Anyone taking blood thinners, particularly alongside **aspirin or NSAIDs**, must be monitored for **excessive bruising or internal bleeding**.

Medical Supervision and Personalized Treatment Plans

Because these drugs are being **used outside of their original purpose**, treatment should always be **personalized** based on:

- **Individual cancer type and stage**.
- **Existing medications and potential drug interactions**.

- **Patient-specific risk factors, including metabolic and cardiovascular health**. Doctors may use **routine blood work, imaging scans, and metabolic assessments** to track how well the treatment is working and adjust protocols as needed.

Balancing Benefits and Risks in Repurposed Drug Therapy

The goal of using **statins, antibiotics, and blood thinners in cancer therapy** is to create a **multi-targeted, low-toxicity approach** that complements conventional treatments. While these drugs have shown **tremendous potential**, their use must be carefully tailored to ensure they are **maximizing effectiveness while minimizing harm**.

As research continues, oncologists and researchers are working to **refine protocols** and determine the safest, most effective ways to integrate **repurposed drug strategies into cancer care**.

Chapter 6: Practical Protocols and Future Directions

General Protocols for Using Repurposed Drugs for Cancer Prevention

Repurposed drugs offer a promising avenue for **cancer prevention**, especially for individuals with **higher risk factors**, such as metabolic disorders, chronic inflammation, or a family history of cancer. Unlike traditional treatments that focus solely on attacking existing tumors, repurposed drugs work by **modifying the body's internal environment** to make it less hospitable for cancer growth.

While research is still evolving, emerging protocols suggest that certain repurposed drugs may be used **long-term as part of a cancer prevention strategy**. These protocols are not meant to replace regular medical screenings but instead provide an additional **layer of protection** for those at risk.

Key Repurposed Drugs for Cancer Prevention

- **Metformin** – Recommended for individuals with **insulin resistance, obesity, or prediabetes**, as it lowers insulin and IGF-1, two major cancer-promoting factors.
- **Low-Dose Naltrexone (LDN)** – May benefit those with chronic inflammation or autoimmune-related cancer risk by modulating immune function and promoting endorphin release.
- **Statins** – May help reduce the risk of **breast, prostate, and colorectal cancer**, particularly in individuals with high cholesterol or metabolic syndrome.
- **Doxycycline and Other Antibiotics** – Could be used intermittently to target **cancer stem cells**, preventing recurrence in individuals with a history of cancer.
- **Blood Thinners (Dipyridamole, Heparin, etc.)** – May help prevent metastasis in individuals with **circulatory issues or clotting risks**, particularly in cancers prone to spreading through the bloodstream.

Timing and Dosage Considerations

For cancer prevention, most repurposed drugs are used in **low to moderate doses** and **adjusted based on individual risk factors**. Some protocols suggest cycling certain medications (e.g., metformin or doxycycline) to prevent long-term dependency or side effects.

Because these drugs work best when combined with **dietary and lifestyle changes**, they are often recommended **alongside metabolic therapies such as intermittent fasting, ketogenic diets, and anti-inflammatory nutrition plans**.

Who May Benefit from a Repurposed Drug Prevention Protocol?

- Individuals with **a strong family history of cancer**.
- Those with **insulin resistance, metabolic syndrome, or obesity**.
- Cancer survivors looking to **reduce recurrence risk**.
- Patients with **chronic inflammation or immune dysfunction**.

While more clinical trials are needed to **establish universal prevention guidelines**, early evidence suggests that repurposed drugs could serve as **a proactive approach** to lowering cancer risk **before it starts**.

How to Combine Multiple Repurposed Drugs Safely and Effectively

While each **repurposed drug** has its own unique anti-cancer properties, **combining multiple drugs** can enhance their effectiveness. However, stacking medications requires careful planning to avoid **overlapping mechanisms, drug interactions, and side effects**. The goal is to create a **balanced protocol** that targets cancer from different angles while ensuring **safety and tolerability**.

Key Considerations When Combining Repurposed Drugs

- **Target Different Cancer Mechanisms** – Using drugs that complement each other is more effective than relying on a single approach. For example:

- **Metformin (targets metabolism) + LDN (modulates immunity)** creates a multi-layered defense against cancer growth.
- **Statins (reduce cholesterol-driven growth) + Blood Thinners (inhibit angiogenesis)** work together to prevent metastasis.

- **Avoid Excessive Overlap** – Some drugs act on the same pathways. For example, both **metformin and statins inhibit the mTOR pathway**, so using them together requires careful dosing to avoid excessive suppression.
- **Monitor for Side Effects and Interactions** – While many repurposed drugs are well tolerated, they may **alter liver metabolism, kidney function, or blood clotting ability** when combined. Regular **blood tests and medical supervision** are recommended for those using multiple drugs.

Sample Combination Protocols

While protocols should always be tailored to individual needs, some of the most **well-**

researched repurposed drug combinations include:

- **For Cancer Prevention:**
  - Metformin (500–1000 mg daily) + Statins (low-dose) + LDN (1.5–4.5 mg nightly)
  - This combination supports **metabolic regulation, immune enhancement, and inflammation control**, making it ideal for individuals at high risk of cancer.
- **For Active Cancer Therapy (with Medical Supervision):**
  - Metformin (higher doses) + Doxycycline (intermittent use) + Blood Thinners (if needed for clotting risk) + Standard Cancer Treatment
  - This protocol targets **cancer metabolism, stem cells, and tumor angiogenesis** while supporting the effectiveness of chemotherapy or radiation.

- **For Cancer Survivors (to Reduce Recurrence Risk):**
  - **Metformin + LDN + Intermittent Antibiotic Use + Diet-Based Metabolic Therapies (e.g., fasting, ketogenic diet, anti-inflammatory nutrition)**
  - Since cancer recurrence is often driven by **dormant cancer cells and immune suppression**, this approach works to **keep the body in a state that is hostile to cancer regrowth**.

Integrating Repurposed Drugs with Conventional Cancer Treatments

For those undergoing chemotherapy, radiation, or immunotherapy, repurposed drugs should be used strategically:

- **Metformin and Statins** – May **enhance the effects of chemotherapy** and reduce tumor resistance.
- **LDN and Blood Thinners** – May **improve immune response** and reduce metastasis risks.

- **Doxycycline** – Can be used intermittently to **target cancer stem cells**, especially after chemotherapy.

Since each drug affects the body in different ways, working with **a knowledgeable medical provider** is essential to **personalize dosing and avoid unwanted interactions**.

As research continues, combining **repurposed drugs, metabolic interventions, and standard cancer therapies** may **pave the way for safer, more effective cancer treatment protocols** in the future.

The Role of Diet, Fasting, and Supplements in Enhancing Drug Effectiveness

Repurposed drugs offer a powerful way to disrupt cancer's survival mechanisms, but **diet and lifestyle interventions** can further **enhance their effects**. Since many of these drugs target **metabolism, inflammation, and immune function**, combining them with **strategic dietary approaches and supplements** may create a **synergistic effect**, making cancer treatment and prevention more effective.

Fasting and Metabolic Therapy

Cancer cells rely on **constant energy and glucose availability** to sustain rapid growth. Fasting and ketogenic diets help **deprive tumors of excess glucose and insulin**, forcing them into a **weakened metabolic state**. When combined with **metformin, statins, or antibiotics**, fasting can:

- **Increase AMPK activation** (enhancing metformin's metabolic effects).
- **Reduce inflammation and IGF-1 levels**, lowering cancer growth signals.
- **Improve chemotherapy and radiation response**, making cancer cells more vulnerable to treatment.

Studies suggest that **short-term fasting (24–48 hours before chemotherapy)** may improve treatment outcomes while **reducing side effects** like nausea and fatigue.

Key Supplements That Support Repurposed Drug Therapies

Certain **nutrients and plant compounds** can enhance the effects of repurposed drugs while providing additional **anti-cancer benefits**. Some of the most promising include:

- **Berberine** – Works similarly to metformin by **activating AMPK and lowering blood sugar**.
- **Curcumin** – A powerful anti-inflammatory compound that can **reduce tumor-promoting cytokines** and enhance **chemotherapy sensitivity**.
- **Quercetin** – A flavonoid that helps **inhibit cancer stem cells and enhance the effects of statins**.
- **Vitamin D** – Plays a role in **immune regulation and cancer prevention**, especially for **breast and colorectal cancer**.
- **Omega-3 Fatty Acids** – Help lower chronic inflammation, improving the **effectiveness of statins and blood thinners**.

While supplements can support **repurposed drug protocols**, they should be used

strategically and under medical supervision to avoid interactions.

Personalizing Diet and Supplement Strategies

Because cancer is highly **individualized**, diet and supplement plans should be tailored based on:

- **Cancer type and metabolic status**.
- **Existing medications and treatments**.
- **Blood sugar and insulin levels**.

For example, individuals with **hormone-driven cancers** may benefit from **low-insulin diets and anti-inflammatory supplements**, while those undergoing chemotherapy may require **extra mitochondrial support** from compounds like **coenzyme Q10 and resveratrol**.

The Future of Integrative Cancer Care

As research into **metabolic and immune-based cancer therapies** continues, the integration of **repurposed drugs, dietary interventions, and targeted supplements** may **offer a new, more holistic approach to cancer treatment**.

Rather than relying solely on **toxic therapies**, future cancer care may focus on **creating an internal environment that weakens tumors and supports overall health**—giving patients more **control over their treatment journey**.

The Future of Repurposed Drugs in Cancer Treatment – New Trials and Discoveries

The field of **drug repurposing for cancer therapy** is rapidly expanding, with ongoing research exploring how existing medications can be **integrated into standard cancer treatment protocols**. While many of these drugs have already shown promise in laboratory studies and small-scale clinical trials, the next step is to determine their **optimal dosing, long-term safety, and effectiveness across different cancer types**.

Current and Upcoming Clinical Trials on Repurposed Drugs

Several large-scale trials are underway to determine the **real-world impact of repurposed drugs in cancer treatment**. Some of the most promising include:

- **Metformin in Cancer Prevention (MILES Trial, 2024–2026)** – Investigating whether long-term metformin use can **reduce the risk of cancer development in high-risk individuals**.
- **LDN in Breast Cancer Therapy (LDN-BC Study, 2023–2025)** – Testing whether low-dose naltrexone can **enhance immune system function and improve survival rates in breast cancer patients**.
- **Statins and Colorectal Cancer (STAT-CRC Trial, 2024–2027)** – Examining whether statin therapy can **slow tumor progression and reduce recurrence rates** in colorectal cancer survivors.
- **Doxycycline in Combination Therapy (2025 Trial Proposal)** – A new study looking at **doxycycline's effects on cancer stem cells** when used alongside chemotherapy and metabolic therapies.

As these trials progress, researchers hope to establish **clear protocols for using repurposed drugs in mainstream cancer care**.

Expanding the List of Repurposed Cancer Drugs

While metformin, statins, LDN, and antibiotics have been widely studied, researchers are now investigating **other existing medications** for their potential cancer-fighting properties:

- **Mebendazole** – A common anti-parasitic drug that may **inhibit tumor growth and angiogenesis**.
- **Ivermectin** – Originally developed as an anti-parasitic, ivermectin has been found to **disrupt cancer cell signaling and enhance immune responses**.
- **Cimetidine (Tagamet)** – A heartburn medication that may **block cancer cell adhesion and improve survival in certain cancers**.
- **Hydroxychloroquine** – An anti-malarial drug being studied for its ability to

enhance chemotherapy effectiveness by disrupting cancer metabolism. These medications, along with newer repurposed drug candidates, represent **the next frontier in cost-effective, accessible cancer treatment strategies.**

Bringing Repurposed Drug Therapy into Mainstream Cancer Care

For repurposed drugs to become part of **standard cancer protocols**, they must go through **rigorous testing and regulatory approval**. Challenges include:

- **Securing funding for large-scale trials**, since these drugs are already off-patent and less profitable for pharmaceutical companies.
- **Establishing clear dosing and combination protocols** to ensure safety and effectiveness.
- **Overcoming skepticism within the medical community**, as most oncologists still focus primarily on traditional treatments.

However, as more research confirms the **benefits of metabolic and immune-based cancer therapies**, the medical landscape is gradually shifting. Integrative oncologists are increasingly **incorporating repurposed drugs, diet, and metabolic interventions** into cancer treatment plans, offering patients more options beyond chemotherapy and radiation alone.

The future of cancer care **may not rely solely on new drugs, but rather on new ways of using old drugs**, in combination with **lifestyle changes and targeted therapies**—leading to **safer, more effective, and more affordable treatment strategies** for cancer patients worldwide.

Final Thoughts – Taking Control of Cancer Therapy with Repurposed Drugs

The exploration of **repurposed drugs for cancer treatment** is transforming the way we think about fighting cancer. Rather than relying solely on **new, expensive pharmaceutical breakthroughs**, the research into **widely available, affordable medications** offers a hopeful alternative. Drugs like **metformin, low-dose naltrexone, statins, doxycycline, and blood thinners** have already shown significant promise in **targeting cancer metabolism, immune function, and tumor progression**.

While these medications are not **a standalone cure**, their ability to **complement conventional treatments and enhance overall survival** makes them a valuable tool in the growing field of **integrative cancer care**.

The Importance of a Multi-Layered Approach

Cancer is a complex disease, and no single treatment is likely to be **universally effective**. The most promising approach appears to be **multi-layered therapy**, combining:

- **Metabolic treatments** (e.g., metformin, fasting, ketogenic diets) to starve cancer of its fuel sources.

- **Immune-modulating strategies** (e.g., low-dose naltrexone, certain antibiotics) to strengthen the body's natural defenses.
- **Angiogenesis inhibitors** (e.g., blood thinners, statins) to prevent tumors from developing their own blood supply.
- **Standard cancer therapies** (e.g., chemotherapy, radiation, immunotherapy) to directly attack tumors.

By addressing **cancer's vulnerabilities from multiple directions**, repurposed drugs can **help improve treatment effectiveness, reduce recurrence risk, and potentially enhance survival rates**.

Taking an Active Role in Cancer Treatment

For patients and caregivers, the rise of **repurposed drug research** presents a **new opportunity to take an active role** in cancer treatment decisions. While oncologists are beginning to **explore these options**, patients can:

- **Stay informed** by following ongoing research and clinical trials.
- **Discuss repurposed drug options with a knowledgeable physician** who is open to integrative cancer care.
- **Incorporate lifestyle and dietary strategies** that align with these drug mechanisms to create **a comprehensive cancer-fighting plan**.

The Future of Cancer Therapy – A Shift Toward Accessibility and Affordability

As research continues to **validate the effectiveness of repurposed drugs**, we may see a future where cancer treatment is:

- **More affordable**, relying on low-cost, widely available medications instead of expensive new drugs.
- **More personalized**, allowing patients to tailor treatment based on their metabolic and immune profiles.
- **More integrative**, combining conventional and repurposed therapies for maximum effectiveness.

While the journey to **incorporate repurposed drugs into mainstream cancer care** is still in progress, the evidence so far suggests that **this approach could dramatically change outcomes for millions of patients**.

By combining **science, strategic treatment, and patient empowerment**, the future of cancer therapy may not just be about **finding the next blockbuster drug—but rethinking how we use the medicines we already have**.

Printed in Great Britain
by Amazon